Heart healthy foods for longevity

Having a healthy heart is very important for everyone. The term "heart disease" is an umbrella that includes a number of heart conditions. It is the leading cause of death among men and women. In the United States, someone has a heart attack every 40 seconds.

This book "heart healthy foods for longevity", informs you about healthy diets or foods that are good for your heart and overall health. Learn about simple, affordable and "everyday" foods you can eat to keep your heart healthy.

1) Whole grains

Whole grains include all three nutrient-rich part of the grains; germ, endosperm and bran.

Many whole grains are good sources of dietary fibre, which we all need. Most refined grains contain little or no fibre. Dietary fibre can help improve blood cholesterol levels and lower your risk of heart disease. Replacing refined grains with whole grains and eating at least 2 servings of whole grains daily will be great for your health.

2) Leafy green vegetables

Many vegetables and fruits are particularly rich in vitamin C and in beta-carote, which is a form of vitamin A. These work as antioxidants in your body, helping to slow down or prevent atherosclerosis by reducing the buildup of plaque from cholesterol and other substances in the arteries.

Leafy green vegetables like spinach are well known for their wealth of vitamins, minerals and antioxidants.

In particular, they're a great source of vitamin K, which helps protect your arteries and promote proper blood clothing. They're also high in dietary nitrates, which have been shown to reduce blood pressure, decrease arterial stiffness, and improve the function of cells lining the blood vessels.

3) Avocados

Avocados are an excellent source of heart-healthy monounsaturated fats, which have been linked to reduced levels of cholesterol and a lower risk of heart disease. Avocados are considered healthy because they are also packed with dietary fibres and nutrients. Avocados may also do wonders for your souring blood pressure levels. Avocados are packed with oleic acid, which can reduce high blood pressure and cholesterol levels.

4) Beans

As well as being protein-rich, beans are high in minerals and fibre, and since it's a plant protein, it's free of the saturated fats found in some animal protein. Eating beans as part of a heart healthy diet, may help improve your blood cholesterol, which is a leading cause of heart disease.

Multiple studies have also found that eating beans can reduce certain risk factors for heart disease.

5) Tomatoes

Tomatoes contains a natural plant pigment called lycopene, which may help lower your levels of "bad" cholesterol, as well as your blood pressure, thereby, lowering your risk of heart disease. (Low blood levels of lycopene are linked to an increased risk of heart attack and stroke). Tomatoes also contains other nutrients like vitamin B and E, and powerful antioxidant properties, which may boost your heart health.

6) Olive Oil

Olive Oil is a great source of monounsaturated fatty acids, which many studies have associated with improvement in heart health.

Olive Oil is also packed with antioxidants which can relieve inflammation and protect the red blood cells from damage, thereby, lowering the risk of heart disease, heart attack and stroke.

7) Walnuts

Walnuts are a great source of fibre and other nutrients like magnesium, copper and manganese.

Walnuts help maintain healthy cholesterol levels and decrease blood pressure, both of which are major risk factors for heart disease. Research shows that incorporating a few servings of walnuts in your diet can help protect against heart disease. Walnuts are also a rich source of omega-3 fatty acids, which is very beneficial to the health.

8) Garlic

Studies have shown that garlic may have positive effects on heart health by preventing cell damage, regulating cholesterol, and lowering blood pressure. Garlic is one of the most powerful super foods available. It's among the top foods that unclog arteries.

Garlic also contain a compound called allicin, which is believed to have a multitude of therapeutic effects.

9) Almonds

Almonds contains a lot of nutrients, minerals and vitamins that are good for heart health. They're also a good source of monounsaturated fats, which is a healthy fat that is good for the heart because they can lower your bad cholesterol and raise your good cholesterol. This therefore means that for those trying to manage their cholesterol, almond is a good choice of diet.

10) Fish

Fatty fish like salmon, mackerel, sardines and tuna contains a lot of omega-3 fatty acids (unsaturated fats), which is very good for heart health and also reduce the risk of heart disease. Studies also shows that eating fish could lower levels of total cholesterol and systolic blood pressure, thereby, improving the health of the heart.

11) Cheese

Cheese can be a part of a heart healthy diet. Cheese contains conjugated linoleic acid (CLA), which is an unsaturated fatty acid that may increase the amount of "good" cholesterol and decrease the amount of "bad" cholesterol.

The belief that "consuming too much cheese is bad for your health" has been found to be wrong by some experts, after discovering that eating diary products does not increase the risk of a heart attack.

12) Dark chocolate

Dark chocolate have been found to be high in antioxidants like flavonoids, which is associated with a lower risk of heart disease. Consuming chocolate in moderation may decrease your risk of coronary heart disease and stroke.

Eating chocolates may also improve blood flow and lower blood pressure, tho the effects are usually mild.

12) Berries

Berries are rich in important nutrients that are good for the heart health. Studies show that eating lots of berries can reduce several risk factors for heart disease.

Berries also help clear the arteries. Berries may help prevent clogged arteries by reducing inflammation and also cholesterol accumulation, improving artery function, and protecting against cellular damage.

Bad habits that affects the heart

As much as we try to eat healthy diets, we should also avoid bad habits that affects the heart. Some common habits that are bad for the heart are;

1) Smoking
2) Staying overweight
3) Drinking too much alcohol
4) Lack of sleep
5) Eating poor diet
6) Being over stressed
7) Lack of regular exercise.

8) Eating too much sugar

As much as possible, these habits should be avoided, for the good of the heart.

These are some of the common foods that are great for the heart. Also note that there are also guidelines to be followed for a healthy heart. For example, regular exercise/ staying active is very good for the heart, also, stoping habits like smoking is important, as habits like this is not good for the heart.

Bibliography: Alot of helpful and resourceful sites was consulted for the writing of this material. Like:

health line, Google, medical guardian.

I hope this material has been very helpful to you. Your heart health is vital and very essential, so it's important you make decisions and choices that will benefit your heart health. You can also get this book for a special friend, as the health of the heart is an important issue for everyone, you never know who you might be saving.

Also, just as an extra tip, if you're struggling with obesity or other weight issues, or you know anyone in this situation, then get this book;

"Healthy foods for weight loss"- by Daniel Adanu

Thank you very much!

Printed in Dunstable, United Kingdom